A Complete Look at Mitral Valve Prolapse Syndrome

(The World's Most Common Heart Murmur)

By: Jim Lowrance © 2010

INTRODUCTION

Mitral Valve Prolapse is a heart murmur found commonly in the general public and can cause heart palpitations, orthostatic hypotension (dizziness upon standing), other symptoms of an imbalanced nervous system and anxiety/panic symptoms. Medical Research studies have found it to be even more common in thyroid disease patients, especially those with autoimmune type thyroid disorders. It is also believed to be about 5 times more common in females than in males.

Many people with MVP do not experience symptoms while those who do are termed as having "MVP-Syndrome". The condition can also cause an imbalance in the "involuntary nervous system" (dysautonomia) and has been associated with Chronic Fatigue Syndrome in some patients who have it.

Interestingly a heart murmur was detected in me as a teen in the 1970s and they diagnosed it at a cardiologist's office as Wolf-Parkinson-White Syndrome, a potentially serious type of heart murmur but over 20 years later at age 38 I had a new Cardiologist rule out my ever having WPWS. I only had an EKG/Stress Test done by the more recent cardiologist and Mitral Valve Prolapse is usually only detected by echocardiogram (ultrasound imaging), which I didn't request, nor was it recommended by the heart specialist.

I knew nothing about MVP at the time but after extensive search online, I realized that this is what I had for all of those years and that I still have to this day. The nervous system related symptoms of the "syndrome" caused by MVP, in fact worsened in my case to some degree with the onset of autoimmune thyroid disease. I at times believe my CFS (Chronic Fatigue Syndrome) diagnosis, which was co morbid to my treated thyroid disorder also has MVPS as a major contributing factor.

It is my sincere hope that this book will help to provide readers with a general education regarding the symptoms, diagnosis and treatment of this very common heart murmur.

TABLE OF CONTENTS (11 Chapters):

CHAPTER ONE

How MVP-Syndrome May Manifest

The following two stories are fictitious examples, written by me – the author, to serve as examples of how one might discover that they are suffering from Mitral Valve Prolapse Syndrome.

Example Scenario One

"I have the Mitral Valve Prolapse heart murmur. My doctor found it after I went to see him suffering with my heart fluttering and skipping. I had experienced irregular heart beats for many years but the day it became severe for me was a day I returned home from a bicycle ride. I was riding on a trail with my daughter strapped in a booster seat on the back and I became unusually out of breath. When I stopped to rest I noticed my heart was beating at an incredible speed which scared the daylights out of me.

It's not unusual for me to get my heart rate to about 160 or 170 when I'm going max speed but on this day I was peddling only about mid speed and my heart was beating at least 200 BPM. Once I rested for a while it slowed to about 80 BPM but started skipping and fluttering about every third beat afterward, so my fear continued and I made an appointment to see my GP doctor. I was lucky that there was a cancellation by someone whose appointment I was able to be worked into.

My doctor questioned me about whether I smoked and I said no. He then asked if I drank a lot of caffeine or alcohol and to this I answered a big YES. I'm a notorious coffee addict and it is not unusual for me to drink 4 to 6 cups a day of strong Columbian dark roast. He listened to my heart and the flutters were obvious, so he sent me home with a pack containing 2 pills that I believe were called Atenolol that helped to reduce my elevated heart rate and it also stopped most of the fluttering beats. He wrote me an order to have a heart ultrasound done the next day and the Mitral Valve Prolapse was found clearly.

He assured me that taking the low dose drug that helped me and that he wrote me a refill prescription for, would help my heart stay regular. He said it was important not to drink more than one cup of caffeinated coffee per day and to eliminate it completely if possible or switch to a decaffeinated brand and that I should sleep regular and keep my stress level down. He also recommended that I stay well hydrated by drinking plenty of water. I continue to exercise but do so, starting at a slow pace and I'm careful not to exceed my tolerance level for physical exertion. So far, these things have greatly helped and I now have only rare symptoms from the murmur. I hope my story helps others to have hope with this condition."

Example Scenario Two

"Back in my childhood I had a heart murmur but the doctor who found it said it didn't sound serious and that I would likely outgrow it. I always had palpitations and funny, fluttery heart beats in my chest but when I became hyperthyroid at age 41 from Grave's Disease the heart flutters starting getting severe and frightening because they were happening about every third or fourth beat of my heart.

I also began to experience serious anxiety symptoms and occasional panic attacks. My doctor ordered blood panels and found I had Grave's Disease a mildly overactive thyroid gland. I've been fortunate because mine was successfully controlled through anti-thyroid medication and so far I do not need my thyroid removed or killed off with radiation.

I was also sent for a heart ultrasound and they found Mitral Valve Prolapse which was the cause of my heart murmur symptoms. My hyperthyroid symptoms are much better but the heart skips are there about a third of the time and can become worse if I drink alcohol or too much caffeinated foods and beverages. I also get very dizzy and sometimes feel faint when I rise from sitting down and I get really short of breath and very tired when I exercise beyond short walks.

I'm on a beta-blocker blood pressure control drug which helps with a lot of this. I also take as-needed anti-anxiety medication when symptoms of anxiousness or panic become difficult to cope with. My doctor says I may never have to have my thyroid removed but that most people do end up having it done because the hyperthyroidism tends to return and becomes difficult to control with drugs alone. I hope in my case this doesn't happen but will keep getting scheduled check ups so that any sign of more hyperthyroidism is hopefully stopped before reaching a point of my needing another procedure done."

MVPS can vary in Symptom-Severity

The preceding two example scenarios are typical of those who first recognize the onset of Mitral Valve Prolapse Syndrome. For some of these people, they knew they had heart murmurs, many years in advance of experience any symptoms from it. Some MVPS patients experience severe, ongoing symptoms that actually become disabling to them but the level of symptoms does not necessarily correlate with the severity of mitral valve dysfunction.

The two fictitious, example-patients described above, would likely be in the area of MVPS symptom-manifestation that would fall somewhere between moderate and severe.

Regardless however of how severe the symptoms of this common heart murmur are, there are treatments and lifestyle changes that are very effective in controlling and in some cases alleviating MVPS symptoms. These will be discussed in this e-book, in addition to further detail in regard to symptoms and diagnosis in the chapters that follow.

Keep in mind if you have dental work done, your Dentist may need to place you on antibiotics for a week or so before having procedures done, depending on whether or not you are experiencing mitral regurgitation and how severe it is (check with your doctor). This is because with some cases of MVP you may be at higher risk for infection and inflammation developing in and around your heart (carditis), after undergoing dental work.

CHAPTER TWO

Basics about Mitral Valve Prolapse Syndrome

There is a common condition of the heart that

causes concerning symptoms in some patients who experience it, called "Mitral Valve Prolapse Syndrome" as previously mentioned. Other patients with the same heart condition do not have symptoms from it and in this case, it is simply referred to as "Mitral Valve Prolapse" (drop the "Syndrome" off the end of the term). Abbreviated, the terms are "MVP" and "MVPS". Both symptomatic and asymptomatic cases of MVP are usually benign conditions in the vast majority of cases, meaning they do not progress into harmful or life-threatening conditions for most patients.

In this chapter, I want to again address MVPS, the type of the heart murmur that causes symptoms. It is also called a "click murmur" due to a clicking sound that can sometimes be heard in the heart, by using a stethoscope and monitoring each beat. The clicking according to medical sources, is caused by the "Mitral Valve Leaflets" becoming somewhat stretched out, so that they are slightly loose or they develop scar tissue on them and become slightly thickened and both of these manifestations can cause them to have a slight vibration-effect, with heart beats. This may also cause mild, moderate or severe "regurgitation" (blood seepage from the valve) that is picked up as a more prominent clicking sound (murmur) with a stethoscope.

Other patients may not have a clicking sound that is as easily heard through a stethoscope but if symptoms being experienced, point to MVP, a more sensitive test may be ordered for detection of the murmur, called an Echocardiogram. This test uses the same principle as a Sonogram that women who are pregnant have done, to monitor the progress of their babies. Sound waves are sent into the area to be observed and they are transmitted as an image onto a screen, so that even the tiniest movement in the heart can be seen. This is how patients with more difficult to detect MVP, can be diagnosed or have the condition ruled out as a cause of their symptoms.

Severe cases of MVP may cause a more severe form of "regurgitation", meaning the blood-leakage from the valves is more significant, when the heart beats. Heart valves of course are supposed to be self-contained, so that blood flows through them without leakage but with MVP-Regurgitation, blood does escape from the valve and this form of the murmur will sometimes require surgery to correct it however, it is a rare form of MVP, with elderly patients being at higher risk for its development.

Following are some of the symptoms that may occur with MVP, placing the murmur into the syndrome category.

- a racing heart (tachycardia)

- heart skips and flutters

- fatigue

- dizziness

- shortness of breath

- anxiety symptoms, including panic attacks

- orthostatic hypotension (dizzy upon standing from a seated or lying down position)

- sensitivities to chemicals (i.e. caffeine, alcohol, tobacco, chocolate and refined sugar)

The chemical sensitivities I list above are triggers that can cause worsening of symptoms in patients with MVPS. The Orthostatic Hypotension, also called "Orthostatic Intolerance", is also classified as a form of "Dysautonomia", meaning a slight deregulation of the "Involuntary Nervous System" (INS) is occurring. Some medical researchers believe that the dysautonomia found in some MVP patients, is what actually causes the syndrome (MVPS) due to the Involuntary Nervous

System playing a major role in regulating heart rate and blood pressure. When it becomes deregulated due to MVP, this is what causes symptoms, resulting in the syndrome. The heart murmur itself may be mild and still result in an array of symptoms and so how severe they are, does not necessarily indicate a severe case of MVP.

In regard to anxiety symptoms found in MVPS, it has been long known that MVP is notorious for causing chronic anxiety and panic attacks and many patients are actually diagnosed with Anxiety Disorders, due to this underlying medical condition. If patients can find control of the symptoms of MVPS through proper treatment and coping methods, the anxiety symptoms will also be alleviated to a large degree, if not completely resolved. More in regard to anxiety symptoms associated with MVP will be specifically addressed in chapters that follow.

CHAPTER THREE

More about MVP Symptoms

Palpitations - If you notice that you have episodes of skipped heartbeats, heart flutters and flip-flops or rapid heartbeats (tachycardia), this can indicate that you have MVPS.

The irregular heartbeats caused by MVPS are due to slight abnormalities in the mitral valve leaflets, or the supporting valve chords, or both. These structures allow the leaflet(s) to prolapse (or buckle) back into the left atrium during the heart's contraction-ventricular systole.

While medical research has not concluded definitively what causes the mitral valve to prolapse abnormally in some people, they theorize that it is due to these valve leaflets becoming either thickened or stretched out over time and this causes them to vibrate or quiver slightly as previously mentioned. This is why it is referred to as a "click murmur" due to the sound it can sometimes make when the heartbeat is listened to closely with a stethoscope.

Anxiety - If you are experiencing panic attacks, frequent episodes of free-floating anxiety or depression symptoms, with no apparent cause for them, this may indicate that you have MVPS, if one or more of the other symptoms as listed previously are also present.

Anxiety is one of the more frightening symptoms of MVPS because panic attacks are the more common type of anxiety that people with this disorder experience. Medical research is not clear as to how anxiety symptoms are caused by MVPS, but some sources state that it could be due to slightly abnormal electrical impulses in the heart, caused by the abnormal prolapsing of the mitral valve leaflets, which triggers the fight or flight response (adrenaline rush) more frequently or at inappropriate and unexpected times.

While anxiety is listed more commonly for MVPS, depression is also experienced frequently in patients with the murmur. Patients may find that they frequently experience both of these emotions simultaneously or they may find that these alternate, so that they are experiencing anxiety at times and depression at other times.

Hypotension - Dizziness in general and dizziness upon standing from a sitting or lying down position (supine) means you are experiencing spells of low blood pressure, low blood volume (hypovolemia) or possibly an ongoing problem with inadequate blood pressure, which can indicate that you have MVPS.

The term for getting dizzy upon first rising, after sitting or lying down is "orthostatic hypotension" and is a form of "dysautonomia," which is a medical term for an irregular response by the involuntary nervous system. This system of the body, also referred to as the "autonomic nervous system" automatically regulates our involuntary bodily functions, such as heart rate, respiration and blood pressure changes with physical activities.

Certain diseases and disorders, including MVPS, can cause this system of our body to operate abnormally, which can result in blood pressure not rising enough upon standing (hypotension) to supply adequate blood circulation to the heart and brain. While this irregular blood pressure response upon standing usually only lasts a few seconds, it can also make a person with MVPS; feel faint, dizzy and pressure-type sensations in the head and neck. This dysautonomia aspect may also be the cause of the anxiety symptoms addressed in the previous subheading, according to some medical sources.

Breathlessness - If you become short of breath more easily and have less tolerance for exercise and physical exertion, this may indicate you have MVPS.

People with MVPS will find that they become fatigued more easily from exercise and physical exertion and that they become short of breath more easily as well. Tolerance for exercise can become noticeably lowered in people with MVPS when they are experiencing the onset of symptoms they have not previously experienced with physical exertion.

This syndrome can have an onset (symptom flares) at any age according to medical sources, however symptoms are more common in women and more commonly found in ages beginning in the mid-teens and older. Some MVPS patients may find that everyday activities fatigue them more easily and more often than before experiencing the syndrome.

Chemical Sensitivities - If you have become sensitive to caffeine, chocolate, alcohol, excess sugar and other stimulants, this may indicate you have MVPS.

People who are experiencing MVPS find that they have unpleasant aftereffects from foods and drinks containing stimulant-type chemicals. Tobacco use can also cause symptom flares. These people will find that overindulgence of these chemicals or that even small to moderate amounts of any type stimulant can cause them symptom reactions.

Even an extra cup of coffee or a chocolate bar can cause their heart to skip beats or flutter and can also trigger anxiety attacks, depression and fatigue more easily. We could also add "stress" to this category because stress is stimulating and a necessary mechanism in our daily lives however, stress levels that are excessive or prolonged can cause the same symptom flares in MVPS patients that other stimulants can.

While a patient will notice the symptoms previously listed, before they suspect that MVPS could be the cause, these are observations that should prompt a visit to a licensed physician. Once a patient has described their symptoms to their doctor in-detail, he can perform a physical, including listening very closely to the patient's heart.

He may detect a heart murmur by stethoscope but in many cases, MVP cannot be detected unless the patient is sent (referred) to a cardiologist/heart specialist for a test called an "echocardiogram." This test uses very sensitive sound waves, transmitted onto a screen, so that the function of the heart can be monitored very clearly. If a patient has Mitral Valve Prolapse, the condition will be detected and definitively diagnosed using this imaging test.

CHAPTER FOUR

More about Orthostatic Hypotension

Normally, blood pressure rises slightly when a person first stands up, which allows blood to be transferred from the lower part of the body, to the upper part of the body. With orthostatic hypotension the blood pressure instead will drop slightly. Some people with this condition do actually pass out but is not common unless a person has a serious heart condition or is elderly. Because of this abnormal and sudden drop in blood pressure, some people with OH will also experience a short term increase in heart rate, referred to as "tachycardia" (beats exceeding 100 per minute without exertion). This is the body's attempt to correct the sudden episode of hypotension.

OH is a common condition that causes the one experiencing it to feel dizzy and/or faint when first standing-up as previously mentioned. Most cases of this condition are mild and not harmful or difficult to treat. In most cases, any actual danger the condition poses is the risk of experiencing injury from a fall, due to becoming dizzy or faint when it occurs. It is also experienced commonly by thyroid patients, especially those with Grave's disease but it can also occur with hypothyroid states when blood pressure and heart rate become inadequate. People with blood glucose problems, such as hypoglycemia (sudden drops in levels), people who are diabetics and those who become dehydrated or anemic, can also experience symptoms of OH.

Orthostatic Hypotension (OH) is a form of dysautonomia. When a person experiences a problem with their involuntary nervous system (INS), the result can be one of a number of conditions that fall under the dysautonomia category, which includes OH. This means that involuntary bodily functions such as heart beat, breathing and blood pressure regulation, become imbalanced due to not being correctly regulated by the INS. As a result the condition may cause a variety of symptoms including orthostatic hypotension.

Orthostatic Hypotension means you experience sudden drops in blood pressure when first standing or a continued worsening of low blood pressure during periods of standing. Other medical names for this condition include "Postural Hypotension" and "Neurally Mediated Hypotension". People with this condition often experience an abnormal drop in blood pressure when standing up from lying down or from a seated position. The INS is supposed to maintain blood pressure with changes in body positions and should actually cause a temporary, mild rise in blood pressure when standing up, in order to move blood from the lower extremities, to the upper part of the body.

There are a number of symptoms that can occur with OH, in addition to those already mentioned. The drops in blood pressure after standing from supine positions usually only last a few seconds, as the blood pressure is normalizing. If this bodily response is mildly, moderately or severely hindered by an imbalance within it, the symptoms experienced may include the following.

• dizziness

• headache

• blurred vision

• nausea

• increased heart rate (tachycardia)

• possible fainting (syncope)

Some people with OH also report experiencing spells of fatigue from this condition, especially after repeated episodes of OH when their activities require a great deal of postural changes throughout the day.

While dysautonomia from MVPS is a common cause for OH, other things that can contribute-to or serve as a cause for an abnormal INS, resulting in OH include other types of heart conditions (including other less-common murmurs), certain medications, dehydration, endocrine diseases (i.e. diabetes, thyroid imbalance and adrenal insufficiency) neurological diseases and low sodium (salt) in the body. Other types of chronic diseases and illnesses that require prolonged bed rest can also be a cause of OH and dysautonomia.

Treatment for OH depends on its severity. Most people have mild cases of OH and their doctors will prescribe a healthy diet, exercise and adequate rest and sleep to help with the condition. In more severe cases, medications may be prescribed to help regulate the abnormal fluctuations in blood pressure. An increase in sodium (salt) intake may be also suggested by a doctor if hypertension is not also present. An increase in fluid intake might also be suggested, to help keep blood volume at adequate levels in the body.

Medications that might be administered to an OH patient might include blood pressure regulating drugs such as beta blockers, mineral corticosteroids (a type of cortisol steroid) and/or drugs that stimulate the nervous system. Other patients may be prescribed drugs such as amphetamines or ephedrine, which help to increase adrenaline levels in the body. The type of treatment is based upon how severely the symptoms of OH are affecting the patient but cases that are mild to moderate can usually be treated with diet modifications and lifestyle changes only.

If you experience symptoms of OH, it is important to make an office visit with a qualified medical doctor to determine the cause and to receive treatment that is best suited for you.

CHAPTER FIVE

More about Treament for Mitral Valve Prolapse

Mitral Valve Prolapse (MVP or MVPS) is a common heart murmur but as mentioned in previous chapters, there are treatments and lifestyle changes that can reduce or eliminate the symptoms significantly in most cases. I addressed the symptoms of this disorder in the previous chapters as well but I will again briefly list those most frequently experienced. The main symptoms of the syndrome can include; *rapid heart rate, heart skips and flip-flops, fatigue, dizziness upon standing, anxiety, depression and chemical sensitivities.*

What are the more common treatments prescribed for Mitral Valve Prolapse when is causes symptoms? According to statistics this common heart condition that affects as much as 20% of the U.S. population, usually requires no medical treatment because most patients do not experience significant symptoms (MVP-Syndrome). For the majority of those who do experience symptoms, they also do not require an actual pharmaceutical treatment but when a Doctor does prescribe a drug, it will often be a "Beta-Blocker" because the drug can help to control a number of symptoms that may be present. This drug counteracts the stimulatory effects of adrenaline (epinephrine) or in other words, it partially blocks some of the effects of the hormone adrenaline, thereby controlling the rapid heart rate, the deregulated blood pressure and the anxiety symptoms.

The diet aspect would be to avoid stimulants in your diet as listed previously that can act as triggers for MVPS symptoms. Also a healthy diet should include lots of fruits, vegetables, nuts and grains (complex carbohydrates) which are always a good idea, as opposed to junk foods (simple carbohydrates) that can only serve to quickly stimulate the body, followed by crashes in energy levels. Also a good multi-vitamin helps the body's systems operate at a more optimal level. MVP patients should also take a "magnesium" supplement – a mineral that helps keep heart function healthy but they first need to have their magnesium blood level checked (or other method of mineral analysis) to see how much they need to be taking and to only take the recommended amount.

Exercise is also greatly helpful in regulating the "Involuntary Nervous System" (highly involved in heart function), as well as the heart rate, blood-pressure and anxiety symptoms. It can also help reduce stress levels that often contribute to symptoms. Exercise can be of more benefit than any other single factor of treatment in many cases but a patient must pace their self and only exercise at their tolerance-level, afterward, slowly increasing the level as they are able to do so. Walking is a great way to begin an exercise program and even if you only increase the distance and/or briskness of your walk over time, the benefits can be tremendous.

CHAPTER SIX

Strong Association of Thyroid Disease to MVP

Some medical research articles state that MVP is a

common finding in thyroid disease patients, which could mean that thyroid disease may be one of several possible triggers for this syndrome or it may aggravate the condition in people who already had MVP, prior to the onset of their thyroid diseases. I have done extensive search and research on this connection and have found no less than five highly reputable research groups reporting on this association. What does this mean for thyroid patients?

The medical reports themselves state that this fact demonstrates the importance for thyroid patients in being tested for this heart murmur. Some of the research states the possibility that MVP also has an autoimmune component to it or that it may be an autoimmune disease itself. While many patients with this heart abnormality do not experience symptoms, those who do are termed as having "Mitral Valve Prolapse Syndrome" (MVPS) as previously mentioned - the syndrome aspect, being a reference to the array of symptoms it can cause.

Some of the symptoms related to this heart murmur, is the result of "dysautonomia", as also previously mentioned, meaning the involuntary nervous system becomes slightly imbalanced, causing a failure in blood pressure regulation and an imbalance in other involuntary bodily functions.

When you have thyroid autoimmunity, this can cause illness, apart from thyroid hormone levels. This is a fact that many Doctors do not seem to recognize because they are of the opinion that until the disease actually lowers or raises hormone levels to abnormal levels, patients will have no symptoms from the disease.

First of all, the thyroid autoimmunity, of itself, causes inflammation in the body. It can also cause goiters and nodules in patients who have normal thyroid hormone levels. Thyroid autoimmunity also causes other illnesses, as stated in reputable research articles. The un-well feeling patients get with thyroid disease, is in part due to the disease itself.

Some patients with highly elevated antibodies may feel un-well even when they are on proper thyroid dose. They may need an anti-inflammatory or supplements like selenium, to help lower the antibodies and their effects. Their thyroid medications over time will also help do this.

There are many research articles, stating the same conclusions, that the thyroid autoimmunity itself is a cause of symptoms. These conclusions, from research conducted over a span of many years, is still unknown or unrecognized by many Doctors. The articles contain such phrases as; "systemic inflammatory reaction", caused by thyroiditis. This means the inflammation is not always localized, only in the area of the thyroid as some Doctors will tell their patients.

My belief is that some patients have more problems with the inflammatory response, than do others. It is a known fact, that inflammation is a cause of fatigue. It also causes our adrenals to remain in overdrive because "cortisol" from the adrenals, is not only the stress hormone but is an anti-inflammatory agent. I feel this is why adrenal fatigue can also be a factor.

It is possible that people who already have MVP but who also experience the onset of an autoimmune thyroid disease (Graves' disease or Hashimoto's thyroiditis), see the MVP/MVPS worsen in symptom manifestations. It is also possible that thyroid autoimmunity itself, serves as a trigger for causing MVPS. These must be considered as possibilities because medical research studies have shown the condition to be very common in thyroid patients, as opposed to control groups (non thyroid disease participants).

Professor Bell, director of the endocrine clinic at the University Of Alabama School Of Medicine in Birmingham, AL has reported finding MVP present in 41% of patients with Hashimoto's thyroiditis and in 41% of Graves ' disease patients who were studied. (Source: WebMD)

Professor M.E. Evangelopoulou and colleagues from Alexandra Hospital at Athens University School of Medicine reported an average of 1 in 4 patients with Graves' and Hashimoto's, as having co morbid (associated) MVP. None of the healthy people in the control group without thyroid disease were found to have MVP. (Study Title: Heart Valve Defect Common in Patients with Thyroid Disease)

The American Journal of Psychiatry published a study in 1987 that states there is strongly confirmed association between panic attacks, mitral valve prolapse, and autoimmune thyroid disorders. (Study Title: Mitral Valve prolapse and thyroid abnormalities in patients with panic attacks)

Several studies are also published on the U.S. National Institutes of Health-National Library of Medicine medical research website. One of the studies states that "the prevalence of mitral valve prolapse is significantly increased in patients with autoimmune disorders of the thyroid gland, when compared to normals and nonautoimmune conditions" (Study Title: Prevalence of mitral valve prolapse in chronic lymphocytic thyroiditis and nongoitrous hypothyroidism.)

Another important aspect to this subject is the fact that thyroid patients, who have MVP/MVPS, may in fact confuse the symptoms of the heart murmur with unresolved thyroid disease symptoms. Some medical sources out there also state that people with MVPS may sometimes be diagnosed as having Chronic Fatigue Syndrome. Another connection regarding CFS is the fact that people suffering the condition often have dysautonomia which is also common in MVPS.

I personally see in this subject of MVP being strongly associated with autoimmune thyroid disease, the importance in recognizing how commonly co morbid some conditions are and the importance in considering these connections when thyroid patients are not experiencing the expected symptom relief from their treatments. Doctors should recognize the need in testing for MVPS in these patients whose unresolved symptoms match those for this common heart murmur.

Medical research conclusions revealing a high incidence of MVP in patients with thyroid autoimmunity have proposed the possibility that MVP itself might be the result of an autoimmune process in the body. The immune system at times will attack organs in the body, once recognizing them as intruders/invaders or foreign tissues. The mitral valve leaflets and/or valves may be the recipients of such an attack but rather than causing total destruction of the valves or the supporting leaflets, it may instead cause the thickening and stretching of them.

Heart tissue is very resilient and can in some cases regenerate areas of damaged tissue, such as that occurring following heart attacks. It may be that an autoimmune attack affects the mitral valves and leaflets over time but does not cause significant tissue destruction in most people with the murmur. The smaller percentage of people who do experience blood leakage from the valve (MVP-regurgitation) may have experienced more autoimmune damage. This is a theory at this point and hopefully future studies in this area will continue to find more answers.

CHAPTER SEVEN

My Book Review of: "The MVPS-Dysautonomia Survival Guide"

As a patient advocate for people with MVP and MVPS, I feel inspired to direct fellow-patients to other quality educational resources. The book I offer a review for in this chapter is just such as resource.

According to this well-written, informative book, mitral valve prolapse (MVP) is believed to affect from between 15% to 25% of the general population and is more common in females than in males. About 40% of people with this mild and usually benign abnormality in the mitral heart valve will experience a mild imbalance in their involuntary nervous system called "dysautonomia." This is the aspect of the disorder that is believed to be responsible for symptoms (syndrome) experienced in some patients with MVP.

The full title of the book is *"The Mitral Valve Prolapse Syndrome/Dysautonomia Survival Guide"* and this is my review. When corresponding with the authors, I made mention that I hear from many thyroid patients who have Mitral Valve Prolapse and the related syndrome and they acknowledged hearing from many thyroid patients with the condition as well. I'm grateful for the free copy of the book they sent me for reviewing.

I finished reading this incredible book, the month of February, 2009 and was actually disappointed when I came to the end of it because it was such an interesting read! James and Cheryl Durante have authored this book, along with John G. Furiasse, MD, a director of a medical center in Illinois that brilliantly covers all of the important aspects of a condition called "Mitral Valve Prolapse Syndrome". This common heart murmur that is not widely recognized by the medical community as being significant but that is gaining recognition with each passing year, can seriously affect those who have the syndrome it may cause.

The authors give a detailed but easy to understand description of Mitral Valve Prolapse (MVP) itself with professional line-art drawings included in the book, to show the reader how the mitral valves in the heart and the mitral leaflets extending from them are affected by this condition. They also help the reader to understand the difference between MVP, which is the condition apart from the symptoms it causes and Mitral Valve Prolapse Syndrome (MVPS), the name used for the condition when it does cause symptoms. The book leads the reader through a description of both the physical and psychological symptoms caused by MVPS and how these can seriously affect the quality of life in those who experience them.

The subject of "dysautonomia", a co-occurring imbalance in the function of the involuntary nervous system is addressed in detail as well in this book, which is believed to be the cause of the symptom aspects of MVP-Syndrome. The physical symptoms that result from MVPS-Dysautonomia are thoroughly detailed, including its affects in causing imbalance in blood pressure regulation and in causing imbalances in both the sympathetic and parasympathetic systems of the nervous system. These systems are also what control the amount of adrenal hormone that is produced in the body and how often it is released in triggering the "fight or flight response" (anxiety mechanism) and how these involuntary systems also calm the body down afterward.

The authors point out that this imbalance aspect of MVPS-Dysautonomia is believed to be responsible for the anxiety problems experienced by those with the syndrome, resulting in panic attacks and other conditions of disordered anxiety. Other problems may result as well, including ongoing and severe (chronic) fatigue, dizziness and exercise intolerance, which when all combined, can seriously affect the quality of life for those who suffer MVPS-Dysautonomia.

We then come to the part of the book that helps MVPS patients learn to cope-with and or even overcome the symptoms of this condition, thereby restoring a higher quality of life to them. A number of patient testimonials about symptom-struggles they have experienced from MVPS-Dysautonomia are included, as well as testimonials of recovery from these symptoms and ongoing positive improvement with proper treatment.

The authors detail medication options for treating both the physical and emotional symptoms of MVPS-Dysautonomia but also describe available therapies, such as Cognitive Behavioral Therapy and Exposure Therapy to help with anxiety disorder and phobia struggles, as well as deep breathing and relaxation techniques. Also discussed in the book are methods for helping those who need help in regaining self-confidence and self-esteem that can also be seriously affected by MVPS-Dysautonomia.

The treatments discussed in the book that include those for both physical and emotional symptoms, includes medications and supplements that are commonly prescribed to treat blood-pressure abnormalities and heart arrhythmias. These are given attention in the book, as well as suggestions on how MVP patients can develop proper exercise programs at a proper pace and tolerance level. Suggestions for diet improvements and avoidance of stimulants are also included.

I, the author of this review, have experienced the symptoms of MVPS-Dysautonomia since my teen years and possibly earlier and I related a great deal to the symptom descriptions contained in this book. I also know that both James and Cheryl Durante authored this book from the perspective of having experienced this condition as well which gives the reader a perspective of MVPS-Dysautonomia they can better relate to.

This book is available in print, through major book sellers.

CHAPTER EIGHT

MVP a Medical cause of Anxiety Symptoms

This common condition that often causes a "click murmur" in the heart has been studied by medical groups and found to be a common cause of anxiety symptoms and panic attacks. Though statistics vary in regard to the number of Americans that have this disorder, a commonly published statistic states that up to 1 in 5 Americans have varying degrees of Mitral Valve Prolapse.

While there have yet to be definitive reasons found for why this usually benign heart irregularity causes anxiety symptoms, there are several theories considered. The most accepted theory is that small, irregular changes in electrical impulses that take place in the heart that are regulated by the involuntary nervous system cause episodes of too much release of adrenaline from the adrenal glands. The heart has many nerve impulses triggered within it that regulate the speed of heart function by interacting with the adrenal glands. With MVP, it is believed that these nerve impulses become irregular so that false signals indicating the need for increased heart rate reach the adrenal glands, causing excessive release of hormone (adrenaline surges).

Anxiety symptoms may include the following.

• apprehension

• worry

• feelings of fear

- rapid heart beat

- hyperventilation

- excessive sweating

- blushing

- trembling

- increased blood pressure

- muscle tension

- an urge to escape

Normally adrenaline is released to change the pace of the heart's beating to compensate for increased physical activity (sympathetic response) or when there is a change in body-posture, such as standing from a seated position (postural blood pressure). With Mitral Valve Prolapse the irregular nerve impulses to the heart trigger these adrenaline surges, causing increased anxiety symptoms.

If you suspect that MVPS could be the cause of anxiety symptoms you are experiencing, the symptoms I've discussed are simply observations that should prompt a visit to your licensed physician. Once a patient suspecting MVP can describe their symptoms to their doctor, he can perform a physical, including listening closely to the patient's heart.

A doctor may detect MVP by stethoscope but in many cases, it cannot be detected unless the patient is sent (referred) to a cardiologist (heart specialist) for a test called an "echocardiogram." This test is a version of ultrasound using very sensitive sound waves, transmitted onto a screen, so that the function of the heart can be monitored very clearly. If a patient has Mitral Valve Prolapse, the condition will most likely be detected and definitively diagnosed using this imaging test.

CHAPTER NINE

Coping with MVP-caused Panic Attacks and Severe Anxiety Episodes

A panic attack is a climax of anxiety symptoms that causes them to be experienced suddenly and forcefully. People, who experience frequent panic attacks, have a condition referred to as Panic Disorder". The following four steps which are often used in different variations of Cognitive Behavioral Therapy techniques (CBT) can help those who suffer panic attacks, to calm their selves when experiencing them.

Remind yourself during a panic attack, that you will not drop dead or lose your sanity.

While panic attacks are the most unpleasant type of anxiety that can be experienced, reputable mental health sources state that they do not lead to loss of sanity, strokes or heart attacks, in otherwise healthy people. Anxiety is a normal mechanism, designed to give the body increased strength to escape danger or to fight an enemy should situations arise requiring the need to do so. It is also designed to help us accomplish urgent or important duties that life might present to us. Panic attacks are an example of this important mechanism, occurring "out of context" meaning they are triggered at times when there is no actual need for the "fight or flight" response.

While this improper timing makes panic attacks extremely unpleasant, they are still a normal response the body is designed to experience without causing injury to the mind or body. The real damage chronic anxiety conditions result-in is restricting some of the freedom and enjoyments of life rather than actually causing mental or physical damage. Reminding yourself of these simple facts, can help diminish the effects of a panic attack and lend toward calming yourself down during one.

Focus on the task you are involved in rather than focusing on the panic attack symptoms.

While this step is certainly easier said than done, with practice, you can learn to divert your attention away from the unpleasant anxiety symptoms and direct your focus more on accomplishing an immediate goal at hand. The triggers that cause a panic attacks can be simple things such as waiting in line to be checked out at a grocery store or walking to the front isle of a theater to be seated.

Other times things that cause panic attacks are of more importance and significance, such as standing before an audience to make an important speech or rescuing someone from a burning home. Regardless of the tasks needing performed, you can practice focusing more on accomplishing them than on the panic symptoms they may be triggering. This will channel your attention toward your energy in performing these tasks, rather than upon surviving the anxiety symptoms that are attempting to challenge you.

If you feel panic symptoms arising while being checked out at the grocery line, you might consider focusing intently on the magazines or other items near the check out stand. When your groceries are being checked out, you might consider mentally calculating the total cost of your groceries to see how close you come to the final tally. If it helps to join in with the clerk in bagging the groceries, you might consider this as a diversion from focusing on anxiety symptoms. Any method that helps you divert your attention and energy into a task rather than focusing on the anxiety is acceptable and you can also make a game out of it, so that you look forward to the gains you will make over time and actually begin to enjoy accomplishing these goals.

Realize that you are not alone in experiencing panic attacks and that they are not a sign of weakness.

Panic attacks are experienced by an estimated 6 million Americans or about 1 out of every 75. Mental health professionals who study anxiety disorders, including panic attacks, have found that people who suffer chronic anxiety, are many times the more creative and passionate people in our society. Famous sports figures including pro football players Earl Campbell and Ricky Williams have suffered panic attacks, as well as famous celebrities including Howie Mandel and Oprah Winfrey. This places people who suffer panic attacks and panic disorder in good company with some of our nation's most ambitious people. By reminding yourself that greatly admired and creative people suffer chronic anxiety conditions, you can also view yourself as among the most creative and passionate people of our society.

Channel your anxiety into a positive and creative process.

Many anxiety sufferers have found that when they feel on edge or as if they are on the verge of experiencing a panic attack, they are also at their most creative and passionate level. By taking that anxiety energy and channeling it into positive actions, you can redirect it away from negative experiences. Rather than running from the anxiety symptoms or attempting to escape from them when they occur, try channeling that energy into creating something you enjoy. If you enjoy sculpting, writing or painting, allow the anxiety to trigger your creative juices into flowing by concentrating that energy into those creative arts. If you enjoy sports, such as soccer, tennis or martial arts, channel that anxiety energy into improving upon your skills and techniques in these areas.

If you are involved in something or in a location where this is not possible to actually practice these pastimes when anxiety symptoms occur, you might attempt to mentally play the sport in your mind or carry a small notepad for jotting down notes on how you can improve in the sport when you are able to play again.

While the following final-suggestion for this step might seem unusual, there is a UK website that recently reported that a PhD Stress Management Expert in the U.S. found that anxiety and stress relief can be experienced using romantic and sexual fantasy as an anxiety diversion technique. In his research, he found that people who conjure torrid fantasies involving romantic and sexual scenarios have found that it helps them to divert negative anxiety responses into passionate imagination, with positive results. I would also add the suggestion that you use your spouse and life partner as the object of your fantasies, which will improve both your anxiety symptoms and your love life at the same time.

These are examples of things that can help to diminish the effects of anxiety symptoms and can also help those who suffer panic attacks, to redirect their anxiety into a positive rather than into a negative direction and outcome.

Treatment for anxiety and other symptoms of MVP may also include beta-blocker medications that help control the effects of adrenaline in the body as mentioned previously and/or anti-anxiety and antidepressant medications.

Types of anti-anxiety medications (benzodiazepines) include the following:

- alprazolam (Xanax®)

- clonazepam (Klonipin®)

- lorazepam (Ativan®)

- diazepam (Valium®)
- buspirone (Buspar®) (this one is a azaspirodecanedione class drug)

Types of anti-depressants (selective serotonin reuptake inhibitors) that also work as anti-anxiety medications include the following:

- paroxetine (Paxil®)

- venlafexine (Effexor®)

- fluoxetine (Prozac®)

- setraline (Zoloft®)

- fluvoxamine (Luvox ®)

The lifestyle and diet changes discussed in previous chapters can also significantly contribute to relief of anxiety symptoms.

CHAPTER TEN

Walking – A Safe and Effective Exercise Choice for MVP Patients

Walking is one of the most beneficial and safe exercises and according to medical health studies on walking for exercise, it can also have mental/emotional as well as physical benefits. It can be an ideal way for Mitral Valve Prolapse Syndrome patients to reduce their symptoms and bring balance to their involuntary nervous systems. The suggestions following below can help you develop a healthy regimen of walking as your exercise.

Stretch your muscles before you walk. When you set out to take a walk, make sure to first do some mild stretching of your leg muscles. By doing this, you lower the risk of hyper-extending or causing cramps in muscles that have not been actively used or that may not yet be conditioned well for exercise. It is especially important to stretch your leg muscles when walking in colder temperatures, which can slightly reduce the blood flow to them and place you at slightly higher risk for causing injury to them.

Warm up by starting slowly and building your walk

to a safe level of exercise for you. The importance of warming up is in the fact that your body needs time to adjust to a change in increased physical activity. Starting off slowly and building the speed of your walk to a safe but beneficial speed is important so that you do not overexert.

A slow build up helps your body to slowly become oxygenated and to have proper blood flow to all of your muscles, so that you experience positive effects from the exercise rather than becoming overly fatigued or causing unnecessary soreness in your muscles. Once your body is better conditioned over time, you may wish to increase the briskness and timed length of your walks as you know your body is able to benefit from an increase in your regimen.

Time your walks so that you do not exceed your tolerance level for exercise. When we exercise, our bodies release hormones called endorphins and these are sometimes referred to as the "feel good hormones" because they cause us to have a slightly high feeling and one of wellness when exercising. This good feeling can cause us to misjudge the amount of exercise we are getting because we may feel we are capable of more than our bodies can actually handle at a given time.

Taking a timepiece along on your walk so that you can time yourself to prevent overexertion is important. Some studies on the benefits of walking suggest taking 20 minute walks at least three times a week and afterward increasing the minutes and number of walks if desired and when physical conditioning allows.|

Take a friend along or listening device, to help you enjoy your walk. Some people find that having an exercise partner helps to inspire them to better stick to their exercise regimen. This is also true when we add any type of enjoyment to the walking experience, such as taking along a hand held or clip-on listening device for playing enjoyable music or inspirational lectures.

It can also add pleasure to your walking experience to find an area with beautiful scenery to enjoy looking at as you exercise. Finding a walking track around a lake or in a park with lots of flowers, trees and other features of nature, can add to your walking experience and actually make you look forward to it each time. The goal is making it a pleasurable experience to walk for exercise rather than making into a chore.

CHAPTER ELEVEN

Understanding Congestive Heart Failure

A Rare but Possible Complication of Mitral Valve Prolapse

Congestive Heart Failure (CHF) is more common in people ages 65 and older but can affect people at any age who have defects or damage to their heart muscles. If can also be a complication resulting from severe cases of Mitral Valve Prolapse, especially in the elderly.

In most patients, CHF has a chronic course but can be reversed in some cases. Even when it remains chronic (ongoing) treatments can be administered to treat symptoms and to improve quality of life for CHF patients. In some cases, fluid may build in a patient's lungs and/or their heart may become enlarged but there are treatments to relieve symptoms caused by complications of CHF.

Symptoms of CHF

The symptoms can vary among individuals, but the ones that are typically experienced may include the following:

- shortness of breath
- wheezing and coughing
- edema in the feet, ankles and/or abdomen

(swelling)
- fatigue
- heart enlargement
- exercise intolerance
- failure in other organs of the body (i.e. kidneys, liver and brain)

These symptoms occur due to a weakening of the heart muscle over time, which causes inadequate supply of blood circulation to the muscles and organs of the body. A resulting effect of diminished heart function out-put, includes a build-up of fluid around the heart and in the lungs due to it becoming enlarged, which also contributes to symptoms.

Causes of CHF

Conditions that cause heart arrhythmias and damage to the heart muscle can result in the development of CHF over time. If a person has a heart murmur or birth defect in the heart, for example, this can cause the condition to develop as they age and especially when they reach their senior-age years.

Heart attacks can also contribute to the development of CHF due to the resulting damage in the heart muscle that causes less-adequate heart function as a person ages. As the heart muscle struggles to supply proper blood circulation output while it is in a damaged or inadequately functioning state, it will often become enlarged as previously mentioned. This is its attempt to allow more blood-flow through the heart valves but is a serious development that can require emergency care.

Lifestyle Treatments for CHF

If the condition is mild to moderate and not causing significant symptoms, a treating doctor might simply prescribe lifestyle changes and intermittent short-term use of a diuretic medication (for fluid retention). These changes in lifestyle might include the following:

• losing excess weight in the body
• regular exercise at proper tolerance level
• a healthy diet
• reduced fluid intake
• removing sodium from the diet (salt – which results in fluid retention)

This type of regimen would be monitored closely by regular follow ups with the patient, to see if the treatment is working or if prescription medications need to be added.

Prescription and Surgical Treatments

Prescribed medications for more severe cases might include beta-blocker drugs to control hypertension, cardiac glycosides to increase cardiac output and ACE Inhibitors to prevent renin released by the kidneys from converting into angiotensin II (a hormone that causes heart constriction).

Should CHF worsen despite prescribed treatments, these worst-case scenarios might require corrective surgery for damaged or malfunctioning heart valves or for stints to be implanted to open constricted arteries. Rarely, a patient will be recommended for heart transplant if they are determined to be an approved candidate for one, meaning they are otherwise healthy, so that their body will not reject the replaced organ.

In many cases, the prognosis for CHF can be good with proper treatment and with close monitoring of treated patients by a qualified MD or cardiologist and as previously mentioned, is not a common complication of Mitral Valve Prolapse.

Severe cases of MVPS, which are also rare, sometimes require surgery to repair the defective valve but for the majority of patients, symptoms are controlled through diet, exercise and natural or prescribed supplements as covered in the preceding chapters. It is my hope that this book has done service in helping to provide a general education to readers, regarding these aspects of this benign but sometimes concerning condition affecting the heart.

(END)